D1433163

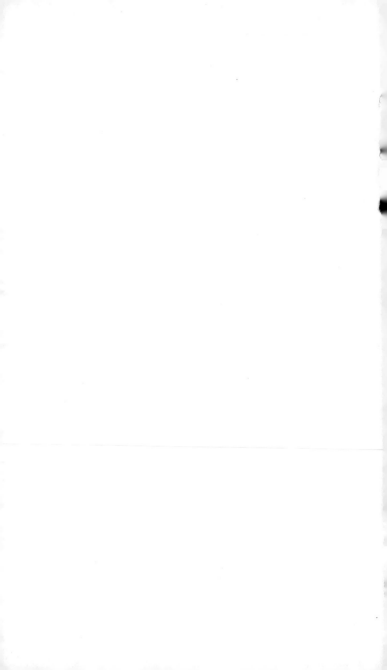

DARWINISM

TODAY

MIND THE GAP

··

HIERARCHIES, HEALTH AND
HUMAN EVOLUTION

Richard Wilkinson

Weidenfeld & Nicolson
LONDON

First published in Great Britain in 2000
by Weidenfeld & Nicolson

A CIP catalogue record for this book
is available from the British Library

ISBN 0 297 64648 6

Typeset by Deltatype Ltd, Birkenhead, Merseyside
Printed in Great Britain by
Clays Ltd, St Ives plc

Weidenfeld & Nicolson

The Orion Publishing Group Ltd
Orion House
5 Upper St Martin's Lane
London WC2H 9EA

CONTENTS

••

FOREWORD

••

Darwinism Today is a series of short books by leading figures in the field of evolutionary theory. Each title is an authoritative pocket introduction to the Darwinian ideas that are setting today's intellectual agenda.

The series developed out of the Darwin@LSE programme at the London School of Economics, where the Darwin Seminars provide a platform for distinguished evolutionists to present the latest Darwinian thinking and to explore its application to humans. The programme is having an enormous impact, both in helping to popularize evolutionary theory and in fostering cross-disciplinary approaches to shared problems.

With the publication of **Darwinism Today** we hope that the best of the new Darwinian ideas will reach an even wider audience.

Helena Cronin and Oliver Curry

MIND THE GAP

···

**HIERARCHIES, HEALTH AND
HUMAN EVOLUTION**

••

CHAPTER I

From Social Gradients
to Psychosocial Pathways

This book is about health and evolution. But it is not about the most obvious links such as the evolution of antibiotic resistance in bacteria or genetic susceptibility to disease in humans. Rather, it is about the socioeconomic factors that make some societies, and some groups within societies, healthier and longer-lived than others. The causes of changes in health over time, of differences in health between countries or between social classes are to be found not in genetic changes and differences, but in environmental change and environmental differences. This book is, in short, about environmental influences on health.

Why, then, is it published in a series on modern evolutionary thinking? The answer is that it is difficult to make sense of what appear to be the environmental causes of population health without evolutionary theory. Health and illness reflect the interaction between ourselves and the

1

environment, and to understand an interaction we must understand both parties to it. We need not only a better understanding of the environment, but also of how we have been shaped by our common evolutionary inheritance. To know whether a ship will ride out a storm, we need to know not only about the storm, but also about the characteristics of the ship such as its stability, buoyancy and the strength of its hull.

It is obvious that our health is affected by factors such as diet; and it would be trivial to point out that vitamins, fibre and so on are important because of the way in which we have evolved. But many influences on our health are more subtle. We now realize for example that some of the most important links between our health and living conditions are psychosocial: that is, many of the biological processes that lead to illness are triggered by what we think and feel about our material and social circumstances. Rather than simply having a direct effect on health, as does, say, exposure to radiation or lack of adequate vitamins, our circumstances also affect health indirectly through their influence on our subjective experience of life.

Our growing recognition of the extent to which people's state of mind influences their physical health demands a lot of rethinking. Evolutionary theory can help this process by clarifying not only why we are sensitive to – and stressed by – particular dimensions of social life, but also why these sources of stress lead to disease. My aim in this book is to clarify why health is so strongly related to social and economic circumstances, and to use evolutionary theory to make better sense of why we are particularly affected by the nature of the social structure and social environment.

Much of the research I will describe was undertaken –

by many different people – in order to understand why people further up the social hierarchy tend to be healthier than those lower down. It turns out that this pattern is partly due to the way in which social structure and social position generate anxiety and stress. Indeed, in rich countries, anxiety seems to be one of the most important pathways linking health to social and economic circumstances. Evolutionary ideas will illuminate why some aspects of our social environment provoke more anxiety and stress than others. They also reveal that the biological processes set in motion by anxiety involve a trade-off between their adaptive advantages and health costs that is likely to have worked to the benefit of our ancestors but now probably works to our disadvantage.

This chapter outlines the picture of health inequalities that is emerging from recent studies. The results indicate that psychosocial pathways have a central role in linking health to socioeconomic circumstances. It has often been found that the smaller the degree of socioeconomic inequality, the healthier the society. In societies where there are small income differences between rich and poor, death rates tend to be lower and people live longer. It turns out that this is probably because more equal societies are less stressful: people are more likely to trust each other and are less hostile and violent towards each other.

Underlying these health inequalities are some intensely social factors that exert a strong negative influence on health. They include the direct effects of subordinate social status itself (as distinct from the effects of the poorer material circumstances that normally accompany it), of friendship, of social networks, and lack of autonomy or control. In Chapter 2, we look at why these factors are so powerful. The discussion shows that they are all related to

3

fundamental dimensions of social reality to which we have evolved a particular attentiveness and sensitivity; that is why they are such potent sources of anxiety.

In Chapter 3 we look at the links that have evolved between psychosocial and biological processes: that is, the links between chronic anxiety and diseases related to chronic physiological arousal. Finally, in Chapter 4, I suggest how the social structure and our position within it can exacerbate our anxieties about how we are seen by others – anxieties that go to the foundations of social life, to our reflexive nature as social beings, and our tendency to see ourselves through the eyes of others.

The theme of this book is the remarkable importance, both to health and to the psychological and social welfare of the population, of the extent to which relationships between us are structured by low-stress affiliative strategies which foster social solidarity, or through much more stressful strategies of dominance, conflict and submission. Which social strategy predominates is mainly determined by how equal or unequal a society is. Income inequality affects everything from the kind of social structure individuals face to the nature of early emotional development. Socioeconomic inequality exerts a profound effect on the quality of the social environment and the psychosocial welfare of the population. Understanding the processes involved throws new light on the politics of class and inequality in modern societies.

Health inequalities

The last quarter of the twentieth century saw a rapid increase in our understanding of the main influences on the health of populations. It is now clear that standards of population health are overwhelmingly affected not so much by medical care as by the social and economic circumstances in which people live and work.

Recognition of the importance of social and economic determinants of health grew largely out of research into the wide differences in death rates between social classes. Typically, death rates are two to three times higher among people lower in the social hierarchy than among those nearer the top. Although these differences are larger in some countries than in others, they are found wherever suitable data have been collected, regardless of whether people are categorized by education, income, occupation or living area. Rather than a simple contrast between high death rates among the poor and lower ones in the rest of society, the usual pattern is a continuous gradient across the whole society, with death rates declining and standards of health improving step by step, all the way up the social hierarchy. In this way, even people who are comfortably off tend to be less healthy than the very well off.

Another almost universal feature of these health inequalities is that they can be found in most of the main causes of death. Yet the extent to which different causes contribute to the overall gradient in death rates differs substantially, even from one developed country to another. For example, heart and respiratory diseases contribute much more to the death-rate gradient in the United Kingdom than in France.

These health inequalities usually account for differences of five to ten years in life expectancy between rich and poor within countries – and occasionally for as much as a fifteen-year difference. Understandably, research into these inequalities has been motivated partly by an interest in social justice, and partly by the hope that the differences will provide important clues to the factors affecting the health of whole societies.

With the initial studies, it seemed possible that these health inequalities reflected a process of selection whereby the healthy moved up the social scale and the unhealthy moved down. However, studies following people from birth to middle age and beyond showed that health-related social mobility makes only a small contribution to health inequalities. Indeed, compared with the non-mobile population who do not change class, socially mobile people tend to diminish the class differences because their health tends to be intermediate between that of the class they leave and the one they join.

Large health differences remain even when studies are controlled for smoking, diet, exercise and other behaviour affecting health. A particularly striking example comes from Michael Marmot's study of office-based civil servants. Death rates from heart disease were four times higher among the most junior (lower-class) staff than among the most senior (higher-class) staff, and most of this difference was left unexplained even after taking into account health-related behaviour and other important risk factors such as cholesterol level, blood pressure, glucose tolerance and height.

Having discovered that these health inequalities were not primarily due to social selection, health-related behaviour or the quality of medical care, most of us working in this area of research assumed that they must be due to differences in material living standards between social classes. It looked then as if our task was to discover the damage done by bad housing, air pollution, poor diet, inadequate heating and other aspects of people's circumstances.

With hindsight it looks as if we were suffering from a remarkably de-socialized view of human beings. We assumed that the key relationships were those between people and things – a belief no doubt strengthened by the economic view that wellbeing depends on individual material consumption. The social aspects were somehow too ephemeral to count beside the concrete environmental problems. Since then, research findings have gradually forced us to see that what matters most, at least in terms of standards of health in modern societies (and probably even for people who still suffer from air pollution and damp housing), is psychosocial welfare and the quality of the social environment. This is not to say that the direct effects of material factors are unimportant; rather, it is to acknowledge that the indirect psychosocial effects of relative deprivation are unexpectedly powerful.

Initially I think that I, like others working in this field, had made an unstated assumption that human evolution was driven almost wholly by the relationship between the species and its natural material environment. The struggle for life was imagined to be a struggle with the natural world, with health as one of the indicators of the success of that struggle. Although the artificial 'built' material environment has today largely replaced the natural environment, there seemed little reason to doubt the continued primacy of the material environment. However, that ignores the crucial importance of the social environment. As the evolutionary biologist Richard Alexander has pointed out, the primary hostile force of nature encountered by human beings is other humans. Conflicts of interest are pervasive, and, to paraphrase Alexander, the competitive strivings of other members of our species become the most salient feature of our evolutionary landscape. By virtue of having all the same needs, other members of our own species are our most feared competitors – for housing, jobs, sexual partners, food, clothing and so on. But they are also our only source of help, friendship, assistance, learning, care and protection. This means that the quality of our social relationships has always been vital to our material welfare. Depending on our relations with others, we could gain or lose the world.

Research into population health provides a re-socialized view of our humanity: it begins to show how we are affected by our social environment. What is at stake is not just physical health but psychosocial welfare too. Nor are these effects simply to do with individual psychology and circumstances: instead there are dimensions of the socio-economic structure that exert a powerful influence on the psychosocial welfare of whole populations.

Explanations

Because a wide range of diseases contributes to the social gradient in health, researchers were initially unsure whether they should be looking for a single 'general vulnerability factor' or for hundreds of different risk factors, each contributing to a higher incidence of a particular disease among those lower down the social scale. Are people lower down the social scale more vulnerable to a set of risk factors to which everyone is exposed, or are some people simply more exposed than others to the same set? Although the answer is inevitably a combination of the two possibilities, the most important single part of the picture, and the part that tells us most about human welfare, concerns the social determinants of general vulnerability.

For many years it was assumed that the psychosocial determinants of health played a fairly marginal role in population health. Although early studies such as those on the influence of bereavement – showing that the death of one partner increases the risk of the other dying soon afterwards – indicated that psychosocial factors could affect health, there seemed little reason to think that psychosocial factors were a major cause of social-status differences in health. Stressful 'life events' such as moving house, divorce, job loss or serious illness of a close relation also seemed to be harmful to health. In addition, there was growing evidence that friendship and social support were good for health, but again it was not obvious that psychosocial factors were powerful causes of health inequalities.

Attitudes began to change with studies of work and of job loss. The amount of control people have over their work was found to be strongly predictive of health (even after controlling for occupational position and other factors). As for job loss, arguments about whether the unemployed were less healthy because unemployment caused illness, or whether it was the unhealthy who became unemployed, hinged on studies of the effects of factory closures where everyone was made redundant regardless of their health. But as well as showing that unemployment leads to a deterioration in health, a series of studies showed that health worsened not only when people actually became unemployed, but also before that – when redundancies first seemed likely and people started worrying about their jobs. This and other findings suggested that psychosocial processes may be important contributors to the social gradient in health.

Among the very different forms of evidence indicating that psychosocial pathways are central to health inequalities, two stand out: the nature of the relationship between income and health in humans, and the physiological effects of social status among animals. Despite the strong relationships between income and health that have been found repeatedly *within* countries, when you look at differences *between* the rich developed countries, you find – at best – only a weak relationship between their average incomes and their standards of health. For instance, even after allowing for price differences, Greeks have less than half the average income of Americans and yet are healthier. Similarly, although life expectancy in most developed countries tends to increase by two or three years every decade, this improvement is not closely related to economic growth: one country's economy can grow twice as fast as another's for perhaps twenty years and yet its citizens may not benefit from any additional growth in life expectancy. Income differences appear to be important within rich countries, but not between them. Even among the fifty states of the USA, where cultural differences are smaller than those between countries, there is (after allowing for differences in income distribution) no relationship between mortality and average state income. Yet within each state there is a clear link between income and health.

The most plausible explanation of this paradox is that what matters to health is not absolute income and living standards, but relative income and social status. Where income is related to social status, as it is within countries, it is also related to health. Where income differences mean little or nothing for people's position in the social hierarchy (such as those between countries), income makes little difference to health. This strongly implies that psychosocial pathways are important: it is hard to believe that relative income is related to health unless those affected have some perception of their relative income or social position.

This view is confirmed by the tendency for more equal societies, with smaller income differences between rich and poor, to have better health. Among the developed countries it is the most egalitarian that have the highest life expectancy, not the richest. There is now a score of reports of this relationship – among developed and less developed countries – as well as an increasing number of reports of the same relationship among regions within countries. In the USA, for example, a strong relationship between income inequality and death rates has been reported for the fifty states as well as for the 282 standard metropolitan areas. In contrast, only two reports have failed to show this relationship and they were based on the same data set; even here, it was only death rates for those over 65 years that did not fit the pattern.

Statistical analysis shows that income inequality affects health independently of average living standards, of the proportion of the population in absolute poverty, of expenditure on medical care, and of the prevalence of smoking.

Societies that are more egalitarian might be expected to have better health simply because the health of the poor is more sensitive to changes in income than the health of the rich. Every £1000 redistributed from rich to poor tends to improve the health of the poor by more than its loss harms the health of the rich, hence average standards of health would rise. But even after taking this effect into account, it seems that there are substantial additional health benefits to living in a more egalitarian society. People on a given level of income, particularly those on lower incomes, seem to be healthier in more egalitarian places. In other words, greater equality is related to better health not only because there are fewer relatively poor people, but also because people over a wide range of incomes tend to be healthier where income differences are smaller. Distinguishing between these two mechanisms seemed particularly important to researchers who assumed that the effects of individual income on health reflected the direct influence of material circumstances, whereas the effects of pure inequality depended on much stranger psychosocial processes. However, because it now looks as if individual income, like inequality, affects health through psychosocial processes, and it makes little difference to policy whether health benefits come by one path or the other, the distinction between the pathways turns out to be less significant than once thought.

Confirmation of the importance of social status to health also comes from animal studies. As we shall see in Chapter 3, experiments in which the social status of monkeys is manipulated show that low social status produces many of the same physiological risk factors for disease among monkeys as among human beings. In these animal studies, the key processes linking health to social status are psychosocial: by manipulating social status while controlling both diet and the physical environment, the studies rule out any obvious material explanations; and observations of the animals' behaviour and physiological arousal, including levels of stress hormones, clearly reveal that low social status increases anxiety. These findings are now underpinned by a growing understanding of the biological pathways that link stress, or chronic anxiety, to the observed physiological changes that put health at risk.

Although income distribution serves as an indicator of both the degree of social hierarchy and the burden of relative deprivation on a population's health, research findings allow us to go a good deal further in understanding the social processes involved in the relationship between inequality and health. In my earlier book *Unhealthy Societies*, I discussed some societies that were unusually egalitarian and unusually healthy: circumstantial evidence suggested that they were also unusually cohesive, as if income differences created or expressed social fragmentation and division. In each case, trends towards greater equality and better health (or less equality and worse health) were accompanied by matching gains (or losses) in social cohesion. One example is the UK during the two world wars, when income differences narrowed dramatically. There was a widely acclaimed sense of camaraderie; and, remarkably, civilian health improved two or three times faster than normal. A second example is Roseto, a small town in Pennsylvania that had a remarkable health advantage over neighbouring towns. Epidemiologists who studied it found that its good health could not be explained by differences in nutritional and behavioural risk factors. Instead, they atttibuted its health to the unusually close-knit community relationships. So confident were they of this explanation that they predicted that if Roseto lost its sense of community, it would also lose its health advantage – a prediction that a more recent study has borne out. Another example is eastern Europe during the 1970s and 1980s when, after rapid improvements in earlier decades, health standards suddenly either ceased to improve or deteriorated – in striking contrast to what was happening in western Europe. These trends were accompanied by increasing inequality, by a growing air of cynicism in public life, by a 'privatization of social life' and by substantial increases in alcohol consumption. As a final example consider Japan, which by the end of the 1980s had achieved the highest life expectancy in the world and seemed a highly cohesive society – the culmination of a long period of narrowing income differences and, almost uniquely in the developed world, of falling crime rates.

Since these initial impressions, new, more testing data have come to light that strongly confirm the tendency for more egalitarian societies to be more cohesive. Among the fifty states of the USA, the proportion of people who feel they can trust others tends to be much higher in states where income differences are smaller. People in more egalitarian states find each other more helpful and are more likely to belong to voluntary clubs and associations. The causal relationship appears to run from income distribution, through the quality of the social environment, to health. There is also some international evidence suggesting that people trust each other more where income differences are smaller.

Other measures of the quality of the social environment show a similar pattern. For example, questionnaires designed to measure how often people had hostile feelings were given to random samples of the population in each of ten US cities. Instead of finding only random individual differences in hostility, the questionnaires revealed that significant differences in average hostility levels between the cities were related to morality. The hostility differences between the ten cities were in turn closely related to the scale of income inequality in those cities.

The close link between inequality and the quality of the social environment is also illustrated by Robert Putnam's 1993 study of local government and the extent to which people were involved in community life in the regions of Italy. Putnam calculated an index of 'civic community' for each region by combining all the data he could find about people's involvement in local community life. He noted that people were much more likely to be closely involved in community life in regions where income differences were smaller. As well as the quality of community life being related to income inequality, Putnam emphasized that where community relations were stronger, people had more egalitarian social attitudes. He writes, 'Citizens in the more civic regions, like their leaders, have a pervasive distaste for hierarchical authority patterns.' Indeed, he even goes as far as to say, 'Equality is an essential feature of the civic community.'

Another important indication of the relationship between equality and the quality of the social environment comes from research into homicide and violent crime. Numerous national and international studies have shown that there is a strong tendency for homicide rates to be higher in countries where there is more inequality. Within the USA, homicide rates in 1990 varied from state to state from 2 to 18 homicides per 100,000 of the population. Much the biggest single influence accounting for these differences was income inequality. A review of thirty-four comparable studies showed that the relationship between income inequality and both homicide and violent crime is robust and exists in many different cultures.

These relationships between income inequality and characteristics of the social environment (such as trust, hostility, involvement in community life, homicide and violence) are strong. Indeed, around half of the differences in the social environment – measured in any of these ways – are probably due to differences in income distribution alone.

Putnam refers to the more egalitarian relationships that foster closer community relations as 'horizontal', and contrasts them with the 'vertical' patron–client relationships that characterized the less civic regions of Italy. This is a useful contrast: it draws attention to the opposition between social hierarchy and friendship and how the quality of social relations deteriorates (with more violence, less trust and so on) as society becomes more unequal and hierarchical. But hierarchy and the quality of social relations are closely related to each other in another important way: it is not just that social relations worsen when societies are more hierarchical – intriguingly, both factors are also powerfully related to health. Low social status and weak social affiliations are among the most important risk factors affecting the health of modern populations. Studies comparing people with low and high social status or those with weak and strong social support networks, have reported two- or three-fold differences in morbidity and mortality rates.

Other risk factors – such as exposure to toxic materials – have been reported to cause bigger differences in death rates in exposed than in non-exposed groups, but in such cases the proportion of the population exposed to significant quantities of dangerous materials is usually tiny and so the overall effects on population health are small. In contrast, a large proportion of the population are exposed to the difficulties of subordinate social status and poor social networks, so the combination of high proportions of the population exposed, and big differences in risk, makes these extremely important risk factors. Indeed, there could hardly be a more harmful mix for population health than widening differences in social status and a simultaneous atrophying of friendship networks. That the two are statistically so closely linked is an additional reason for believing that the relationship between income distribution and health is indeed causal: given that wider income differences increase the burden of relative deprivation or low social status and are accompanied by a simultaneous atrophying of social relations, it would be extraordinary if health did not suffer as income differences widened.

We are still some way from achieving a generally accepted view of how social status, friendship and cohesion exert such a powerful influence on health. It seems hard to explain why they should be so closely related to health. Why does friendship matter so much? And why should differences in social status have such an effect on health if – as the monkey experiments suggest – it is not through material factors such as housing and diet? Increasingly, standards of population health in the developed world are dominated by a range of psychosocial variables that seemed inexplicably important to health. These include how much control people actually have, or feel they have, over work and over other areas of life; a perceived 'imbalance' between the emotional efforts and rewards people put into, and get out of, their work; having to cope with stressful 'life events' or 'ongoing difficulties'; poor attachment and emotional difficulties early in life that can cast a long shadow over health in later life; and 'negative social relationships' such as marital conflicts. Together with the health risks of external social factors such as these, there is a growing body of evidence that the kind of psychological states likely to accompany them – such as a sense of helplessness, low self-esteem, hostility, hopelessness, depression and low 'life satisfaction' – are also predictive of poor health.

There are still those who prefer to believe in the primacy of direct material influences on health. They suggest that friends may be important for the material support they give each other. But in modern societies few friends give each other enough material support to make a real difference to living conditions. How many poor people have friends who would pay off their rent arrears or provide long-term income supplements? What they more commonly give each other are alcoholic drinks, cigarettes, the proverbial 'cup of sugar' that neighbours are said to lend each other, minor infections and, more recently, perhaps AIDS. Even where friends give each other nothing worse than unnecessarily large dinners and an occasional bed for the night, the mix is of no obvious benefit to health.

One might argue that causality could work the other way round too: for example, instead of social isolation causing poor health, prior ill-health might reduce social contact and friendship. However, these possibilities are ruled out by studies that exclude people with pre-existing symptoms and follow subjects up over time.

In drawing attention to the most plausible psychosocial pathways contributing to health inequalities and to the socioeconomic determinants of health more widely, it is worth emphasizing that these explanations do not represent a descent into the individualistic perspectives and remedies normally associated with personal psychological difficulties. What makes the difference is that the quality of the social environment differs *systematically* from one place to another and that an important part of this variation is linked to structural factors such as differences in income inequality.

The relationship between income inequality and mortality discussed in this chapter have been found internationally in both rich and poor countries, as well as in comparisons of areas within countries. Health is likely to be affected because the social environment deteriorates in societies where income inequalities are greater. The relationships are robust and seem not to be confined to particular cultures: in addition to the data from within the USA and Italy, the relationship between income inequality and homicide has been found repeatedly in international studies as well as in studies within single countries. The evidence from many different societies suggests that there are powerful structural influences on the psychosocial welfare of populations.

To understand why psychosocial factors are so closely related to health, we must understand both the psychosocial and the biological processes involved. In Chapter 2 we will get to grips with our psychological sensitivity to social status and friendship.

CHAPTER 2

••

Behind the Social
Risk Factors

In Chapter 1 we saw that death rates tend to be higher in countries and regions where income differences between rich and poor are larger. We also saw that greater income inequality seems to be accompanied by more violence, less trust, more hostility and less involvement in community life. Death rates usually seem to be more closely related to these aspects of the social environment than to income inequality itself.

The statistical realtionships suggest that the pathway from income inequality to health goes from income distribution, through the social environment, to mortality. But the close relationship between death rates and trust, or between death rates and average hostility, does not mean that it is either the lack of trust or the hostility itself that does the damage on its own. Instead, each of these measures probably indicates the nature of social interactions more generally. Rather than regarding any single measure of the social environment as important to health or uniquely related to income inequality, it would be more accurate to think of the different measures of the social environment as highly correlated. So in areas where people trust each other less, rates of violence are likely to be higher and people are less likely to be involved in community life.

Indeed, it looks as if each of these measures tells us something about the overall distributions of social interactions in a society. Within every society relationships will vary, from the most supportive and kindly at one extreme, to the most aggressive and violent at the other. From this point of view, measures taken at any point in such a distribution, whether of trust, domestic conflict or homicide, would indicate the character of the whole of that distribution. We should not therefore regard homicide as a bizarre form of behaviour, unrelated to the lives of most of the population of a society in such a way that the close relationship between the distribution of homicide and the distribution of other causes of death appears inexplicable. Rather, we should see an increased homicide rate as indicating greater aggression and violence on the streets in general; and given what we know of the links between domestic violence in childhood and violence in early adulthood, it may indicate more domestic conflict as well.

As we have seen, social status and supportive social relationships are linked not only because they both exert a powerful influence on health but also because of the strong tendency for social relationships to weaken as the social structure hierarchy becomes more hierarchical. In an important sense, social status and friendship are the opposite sides of the same coin. Social hierarchy, like pecking orders and dominance hierarchies among animals, is based on power, coercion and access to resources regardless of the needs of others. In contrast, friendship is marked by reciprocity, mutuality, sharing and a recognition of others' needs. Status and friendship are therefore two opposite ways in which human beings can come together: on the basis of power in structures of dominance and subordination, or on the basis of social obligations and mutuality.

These principles go to the heart of the two distinct types of social organization found among both human and non-human primates: those based on power and dominance ('agonic') and those based on more egalitarian cooperation ('hedonic'). Since class societies have been predominant throughout human history, we tend to take the agonic forms of social organization as the human norm. But this overlooks the evidence that during our hunter-gatherer prehistory – the vast majority of human existence – we lived in hedonic groups. Anthropologists have described modern hunter-gatherer societies as 'assertively' egalitarian. In a review of more than a hundred anthropological accounts covering twenty-four recent hunter-gatherer societies spread over four continents, David Erdal and Andy Whiten concluded that these societies were characterized by 'egalitarianism, co-operation and sharing on a scale unprecedented in primate evolution':

> They share food, not simply with kin or even just with those who reciprocate, but according to need even when food is scarce ... There is no dominance hierarchy among hunter-gatherers. No individual has priority of access to food which . . . is shared. In spite of the marginal female preference for the more successful

hunters as lovers, access to sexual partners is not a right which correlates with rank. In fact rank is simply not discernible among hunter-gatherers. This is a cross-cultural universal, which rings out unmistakably from the ethnographic literature, sometimes in the strongest terms.

Erdal and Whiten suggested that the egalitarianism of these societies resulted from what they called 'counter dominance strategies'. Just as non-human primates in dominance hierarchies will form social alliances to depose a leader or to defend their own position, so might early human societies have functioned as an alliance of everyone against anyone who tried to take a dominant position. The overwhelming predominance of the exchange of gifts in these and early agricultural societies is an indication of the importance of investment in social relationships. Because other people have the potential to become anything from the most feared rivals and competitors to the greatest source of love and assistance, each person's welfare and safety depended on how they managed their social relations – on keeping other people sweet.

Although massive investments in social relations – in the form of gifts and sharing – were obviously the appropriate social strategy in egalitarian societies where reciprocity was the norm, in a dominance hierarchy such generosity risked exploitation. The use of dominance strategies in an egalitarian social context would, on the other hand, risk exclusion from the cooperative group.

There are many reasons for thinking that friendship is inherently egalitarian. After all, if someone withholds his or her plentiful resources from meeting the pressing needs of a friend, that clearly shows the limits of their friendship.

23

Studies reveal how friendships cope with the strains created when inequality enters the relationship as a result of changes in the fortunes of one or other partner. Recognizing the egalitarian nature of friendship, Plato said: 'How correct the old saying is, that "equality leads to friendship"! It is right enough and it rings true.' The connection between friendship and equality is taken very much for granted. Indeed, in the Cambridge scale for classifying occupations according to social status, friendships are used as an indicator of equal social status. To arrive at this scale, sampled people are asked to state their own occupation and the occupation of six friends. The occupations that turn out to be linked by many friendships are classified as being of similar social status, whereas occupations linked by few are treated as socially distant from each other.

It might seem that the antipathy between friendship and inequality provides an adequate explanation of the tendency for more unequal societies to have a more hostile and less hospitable social environment. But if we think of the distribution of violence – as the most visible sign of a less cohesive social environment – it is clear that violence is not primarily between rich and poor. Except perhaps in revolutionary situations, violence is concentrated in poor areas and occurs primarily among the poor themselves. This is partly because what counts as violence are those forms of coercion not sanctioned by social institutions: making people homeless by ending a tenancy is not an act of violence, whereas hitting the landlord or snatching a handbag is. Inevitably, the effects of 'institutional violence' (non-violent legal coercion) are concentrated at the bottom of society.

In an important sense poverty is, as Gandhi remarked, the worst form of violence. Nevertheless, it is worth trying to understand why inequality is related to the overt physical violence between individuals that is most common in the poor inner-city areas. A strong link between inequality and violence is one of the reasons for thinking that the social environment deteriorates where income differences are larger. Not only is there a close association between inequality and violence, but areas with high levels of violence also have high death rates from causes other than violence. So if we understood the link between violence and inequality, we might well also understand the link between health and inequality.

What clues can the literature on criminal violence give us as to why violence – very predominantly male violence – is more common where there is more inequality? On the face of it, violent incidents often seem to be triggered by seemingly trivial issues, but deep down they are actually to do with people feeling they have been *disrespected*. James Gilligan has enormous knowledge of violence and of violent men. A prison psychiatrist for twenty-five years, he became director of the Center for the Study of Violence at Harvard. In his book *Violence: Our Deadly Epidemic and Its Causes*, he repeatedly shows that violence is linked to the experience of shame and humiliation. Given his enormous first-hand knowledge, it is remarkable that he goes as far as to say, 'I have yet to see a serious act of violence that was not provoked by the experience of feeling shamed and humiliated, disrespected and ridiculed, and that did not represent the attempt to prevent or undo this "loss of face" – no matter how severe the punishment.' As an example, he describes a prisoner who was continuously being punished for his violence and asking him: 'What do you want so badly that you sacrifice everything else in order to get it?' Gilligan recalls that the prisoner

> replied with calm assurance, with perfect coherence and even a kind of eloquence: 'Pride. Dignity. Self-esteem.' And then he went on to say, again more clearly than before: 'And I'll kill every mother-fucker in that cell block if I have to in order to get it! My life ain't worth nothin' if I take somebody disrespectin' me and callin' me punk, asshole, faggot, and goin' Ha! Ha! at me . . . If you ain't got pride, you got nothin'. That's all you got! I've already got my pride.' He explained that the other prisoner was 'tryin' to take that away from me. I'm not a total idiot. I'm not a coward. There ain't nothing I can do except snuff him. I'll throw gasoline on him and light him.'

The central importance of disrespect is confirmed in autobiographical accounts from men who have served time for violent offences. Nathan McCall, a *Washington Post* reporter who grew up in a poverty-stricken neighbourhood in Virginia and served time in prison for violent crime, says in his autobiography:

> For as long as I can remember, black folks have had a serious thing about respect. I guess it's because white people disrespected them so blatantly for so long that blacks viciously protected what little morsels of self-respect they thought they had left. Some of the most brutal battles I saw in the streets stemmed from seemingly petty stuff . . . But the underlying issue was always respect. You could ask a guy, 'Damn, man, why did you bust that dude in the head with a pipe?' And he

might say, 'The motherfucka disrespected me!' That was explanation enough. It wasn't even necessary to explain how the guy had disrespected him. It was universally understood that if a dude got disrespected, he had to do what he had to do. It's still that way today. Young dudes nowadays call it 'dissin'.

Violence has always been one way in which men have tried to 'defend their honour' and prevent loss of face. This explains why it occurs most frequently among those at the bottom of the social scale, is strongly related to income inequality, and tends to be triggered by situations in which people feel their dignity is threatened. Wider income differences mean that more people are excluded from the jobs and incomes that are the usual sources of status. Imputations of inferiority are likely to make people much more sensitive to issues of respect and dignity. Indeed, the fact that violent crime but not property crime is related to inequality (at least as measured among the fifty states of the USA) indicates that what matters most about relative deprivation is not so much the lower living standards in themselves, but the affront to dignity and respect, and the imputation of inferiority that accompanies relative poverty.

Because access to resources is such an important indicator of status, poverty has tended to be defined not just in terms of absolute material standards but also in terms of the minimum standards required to maintain basic standards of decency and human dignity relative to the rest of society. Adam Smith, recognizing the importance of the social connotations of difference in material living standards, defined poverty in explicitly relative terms. In *The Wealth of Nations* he writes, 'By necessities I understand not just commodities which are indispensably necessary for the support of life, but whatever the custom of a country renders it indecent for creditable people, even of the lowest order, to be without.'

Karl Marx also recognized that social comparisons are fundamental to our perception of our circumstances. In *Wage Labour and Capital* he wrote:

> A house may be large or small; as long as the surrounding houses are equally small it satisfies all social demands for a dwelling. But if a palace arises beside the little house, the little house shrinks to a hovel . . . [and] . . . the dweller will feel more and more uncomfortable, dissatisfied and cramped within its four walls.

The role of disrespect and inequality in producing violence indicates our extraordinary sensitivity to social status. Indeed, in hierarchical social settings, human beings seem – overtly or covertly – highly attentive and sensitive to issues to do with status. Imputations of inferiority are highly aversive; and, even when it does not lead to violence, the sense of being put down or ignored generates strong feelings of angst in most of us. Few can remain aloof and suffer such slights with equanimity, even if from any other point of view what was at stake was trivial – ask any professional woman who has been mistaken for a secretary, told to get the coffee, or had her suggestions ignored until repeated by a man. To some extent we have become aware of these issues in the context of race and sex, but 'classism' remains rampant.

Among our pre-human ancestors, position in the dominance hierarchy conferred direct and substantial reproductive advantages: reproductive success was increased both because high-status males had increased sexual access to females and because of the improved survival chances of the young of higher-status females who had better access to food and offered more effective protection. On this basis it would be surprising if sensitivity and attentiveness to social status, the attraction of high status and the aversiveness of low social status, were not all part of our common human inheritance. (The tendency for dominant male animals to partly or wholly exclude subordinate males from breeding may partly explain why men are so much more likely than women to respond to disrespect and insinuations of inferiority with violence.) Yet even if this sensitivity to social dominance is an inherent human characteristic, our long prehistoric existence in highly egalitarian hunter-gatherer societies shows that hierarchical social organization is not an inevitable feature of human society – far from it. Indeed, the organization of our social environment as a dominance hierarchy may have profound – and often undesirable – effects on our behaviour and the quality of our social relations. The egalitarianism of hunter-gatherer societies, which – although recent in evolutionary terms – has been the pattern for almost all of our past existence as 'anatomically modern' human beings, should perhaps be seen as a strategy that avoided the social costs of inequality.

It is not just at the bottom of the heap that people are attentive to social position. Even as early as the late eighteenth century Adam Smith believed that the main driving force of economic activity was people's desire for what he called 'regard'. In his *Theory of Moral Sentiments* he asks:

What is the end of avarice and ambition, of the pursuit

> of wealth, of power and pre-eminence? Is it to supply
> the necessities of nature? The wages of the meanest
> labourer can supply them . . . What are the advantages
> which we would propose to gain by that great purpose
> of human life which we call bettering our condition?
> To be observed, to be attended to, to be taken notice of
> with sympathy, complacency, and approbation, are all
> the advantages which we can propose to derive from it.

Several modern empirical studies have shown that although people's satisfaction with their income is not related to its absolute level, it is related to how it compares with the incomes of others. Most recently Robert Frank in *Luxury Fever* and Juliet Schor in *The Overspent American* have expanded on this theme by arguing that escalating standards of consumption are driven by processes of social comparison including both the defensive desire to maintain respectability and the desire to improve one's status. Schor argues that during the 1980s and 1990s, when income differences in the USA widened, millions of Americans felt poorer despite actually having more in absolute terms. She describes how people used to aspire to an income only about 20 per cent above what they actually had, but as income differences widened during these two decades, the 'aspiration gap' also widened. Survey data suggested that the incomes to which people aspired more than doubled between 1986 and 1994. As a result savings declined and debt increased. The contribution of processes of social comparison in driving these trends was indicated by the finding that the more television people watched, the more they spent and the less they saved. As Schor says, 'We live with high levels of psychological denial about the connection between our buying habits and the social statements they make.'

The French sociologist Pierre Bourdieu has done much to unmask the way in which social status influences consumption. His work shows that an important influence on aesthetic taste across a broad sweep of cultural life is the desire to express and maintain social class distinctions. In one area of aesthetic judgements after another, the higher classes express preferences for whatever is less immediate, less available, less obvious and more difficult, so differentiating themselves from the popular taste of lower classes with remarkable consistency.

Snobbishness is another of the extraordinarily pervasive indications of our concern about social status. At its worst, it causes people to shun, deny or hide their connections with anything that smacks of lower social status, while dropping names and parading their familiarity with all the cultural indicators of higher status.

The causes of the well-known phenomenon of 'white coat hypertension' – the tendency for many people's blood pressure to be higher than usual when measured by a doctor – is often treated as a mystery. But it is merely another indication of our extreme sensitivity to differences in social status. Social psychologists have shown that people's blood pressure tends to increase when they are interviewed by a higher-status interviewer but not when interviewed by an equal or lower-status interviewer. This lends credence to Ralph Waldo Emerson's claim that ''Tis very certain that each man carries in his eye the exact indication of his rank in the immense scale of men, and we are always learning to read it.'

People are sometimes puzzled about what the connection is between dominance hierarchies among non-human primates and social class hierarchies in human societies. Despite their differences, the simple answer is that they are both systems based on what Paul Gilbert called 'resource holding power': that is, power to hold or gain access to resources. This is why relative income and material inequality are such powerful social indicators. The social hierarchy is basically still a pecking order. Despite the myriad of different cultural and social embellishments, the great issue underlying social dominance has always been access to resources, including reproductive opportunities.

By contrast, sharing and gift-giving remind us that friendship is rooted in an agreement not to compete for resources. The gift symbolizes that people have chosen to eschew competition for the necessities of life in preference for relations of mutuality. Sharing food carries the same symbolism where it matters most: over the most basic necessities of life. The continued importance of these symbols even in market societies is shown by the fact that even if you offered to repay your host for a postage stamp you had asked for, you would never suggest paying for the food you had consumed as a guest at dinner.

However, friendship is not only about avoiding competition for resources: alliances in which others come to your assistance, particularly in disputes, are also a resource in themselves. Where dominance hierarchies exist among non-human primates, social alliances are an important source of protection. As Alison Jolly points out, mutual grooming is 'the social cement of primates from lemur to chimpanzee', and it may create social bonds that involve reciprocity. When facing an attack, an animal is more likely to receive aid from animals it has recently groomed than from others. Such alliances also help animals to maintain or improve their position in the social hierarchy. Once again, there are reasons for thinking that strong selective pressures have endowed us with a desire for friendship and a tendency to find rejection or a lack of friends a source of anxiety.

It is the principle of reciprocity that makes cooperative relationships a workable basis of social life. The sense of indebtedness, of the need to make a return gift, appears to be universal and is probably an evolved predisposition that amounts almost to a genetically encoded basis for a social contract. In a world where people's daily survival depended not on money in the bank but on the strength of their social bonds, social exclusion would inevitably be highly aversive. If you are excluded from the cooperative group, you risk being victimized or preyed upon.

Social status cannot be readily defined. Rather, it comprises the characteristics of social groups that indicate dominance and subordination. Although wealth and power are of the essence, other attributes will differ from one type of society to another.

CHAPTER 3

••

The Biology of
Chronic Stress

We now turn to the biological explanations of how psychosocial processes influence health. As Chapter 2 was concerned primarily with sociological processes, we shall start by looking at the effects of these processes on individuals.

Take, for example, the influence of friendship or social affiliations on health. Many studies demonstrate that rates of death or illness are two to four times higher among those who are more socially isolated. In one experiment people were given nasal drops containing cold viruses. Those with friends in few areas of life were more than four times as likely to develop colds as people with friends in many areas of life. Another study found that after suffering a heart attack, people with good social support are three times as likely to survive as those without. Experiments in which monkeys were socially isolated showed that they are affected in much the same way as socially isolated humans.

One of the main conceptual breakthroughs in understanding the socioeconomic gradient in human health came from studies of the dominance hierarchy among wild baboons and captive cynomolgus macaque monkeys. Among the wild baboons, it was possible to see whether social position affected health or health affected social position by looking at what happened when the dominance hierarchy was disrupted or when animals joined a different troop in which they had a different social status. Among the captive monkeys, social status was experimentally manipulated: low-status animals were taken from several different groups and put together in the same compound, and high-status animals were similarly taken from different groups and put together, so that some high-status animals would have to become low status and some low-status animals would become high status. Here it was possible to control diet and hold the environment constant. So any physiological changes could be directly attributed to the effects of position in the dominance hierarchy.

The huge differences in the lives of people and animals make us rightly wary of inferring too glibly about people from what we know about animals. But the similarity between many of the physiological changes associated with low-status among humans and non-human primates demands that we treat seriously the possibility that they might have similar causes. The physiological effects of low social rank were observed in monkeys even in the complete absence of the plethora of differences in socioeconomic circumstances found among humans. The

35

effects cannot therefore be attributed to jobs, housing, smoking, diet, debt, unemployment or whatever. So rather than being linked to social status only indirectly, through such socioeconomic factors, the effects appear to be due to the direct, or 'pure', effects of social status.

Of the physiological changes measured so far, it has been found that subordinate monkeys and low-status humans share a much faster build-up of atherosclerotic plaque in their coronary arteries; are more likely to suffer from central obesity (fat around the waist is more closely linked to heart disease than fat around the hips); have potentially more damaging levels of high-density blood fats relative to low-density blood fats; are more likely to be resistant to insulin; and tend to have raised resting levels of cortisol (a stress hormone) and a less dramatic cortisol response to short-term stress. The low-status monkeys often show behavioural signs of depression and seem to be in a state of almost permanent anxiety and insecurity as they try to keep out of the way of their superiors.

In addition to low status, lack of friends and limited social contact, other psychosocial risk factors are important, including lack of adequate control over work or home life, and emotional difficulty in early childhood, which seems to be a precursor of poorer health in later life. Why are these particular features of life such good predictors of ill-health and premature death?

Initially it looked as if there might be a set of specific psychological states that were damaging to health. However, later work on the physiological effects of chronic anxiety suggest that almost any frequent state of prolonged arousal would be damaging to health. Most of the main psychosocial influences on health can be seen as sources of stress that are likely to cause physiological arousal. 'Life events' such as divorce, forced job change and criminal prosecution are often singled out as stressful. If you feel in control of work and home life, then perhaps there are fewer threatening events imminent that you might be unable to cope with. On the other hand, risk factors such as job or housing insecurity represent the opposite of being in control: they are major threats over which you have little or no control. Friends and supportive social relationships can also be seen as providing opportunities for reducing stress.

What are the main biological processes through which chronic anxiety leads to ill-health? The central mechanisms are part of the 'fight or flight' response. To paraphrase the biologist Robert Sapolsky, in brief emergencies the body mobilizes energy for muscular activity. Physiological processes not essential for producing a faster, more effective response to an immediate – perhaps life-threatening – danger are 'put on hold'. When survival depends on alertness, reaction times and the ability to run fast, all the biological 'housekeeping' functions such as tissue maintenance and repair, immunity, growth, digestion and reproductive processes can be left until later. When the emergency is over, presumably after a successful fight or flight usually lasting no more than a few minutes, nothing is lost as a result of the brief diversion of resources. But when the anxiety and arousal go on for weeks, months or years, the health costs start to accumulate. So broad is the range of possible health consequences that the costs have been likened to rapid ageing and would provide the 'general vulnerability factor' that Michael Marmot and others thought might lie behind health inequalities. This is an important point. Instead of thinking of health simply in terms of exposure to infectious agents or other environmental hazards, we should think more about what affects the body's defences, its immune system and ability to withstand exposure to, or repair damage resulting from, a wide range of potentially harmful circumstances.

The main biological pathways involved are common to most mammals. In a process triggered by perceptions of danger or threat, the body is prepared for fight or flight by both the nervous system and the endocrine system (which secretes hormones directly into the bloodstream). As its name suggests, the autonomic nervous system controls many of the biological processes that take place automatically and is quite distinct from the nervous connections that allow us conscious control over our muscular activity and movement. It has two main branches: the sympathetic and the parasympathetic. The sympathetic nervous system is linked to all the major organs as well as comprising a fine network of nerves supplying blood vessels, sweat glands and so on. When activated, the system causes the release of adrenaline and noradrenaline (epinephrine and norepinephrine in US usage), which contribute to the body's arousal and activation. Adrenaline is secreted into the bloodstream by the adrenal glands, and noradrenaline is produced at all the other sympathetic nerve endings. It is this almost instantaneous response from the sympathetic nervous system that leaves you tingling after a sudden shock such as a 'near miss' when driving.

The role of the parasympathetic nervous system is very different. It is activated during sleep and in periods of relaxation when it promotes energy storage, digestion, growth and what Sapolsky refers to as 'other optimistic processes'. The sympathetic nervous system increases the heart rate and diverts blood to the muscles, whereas the parasympathetic nervous system slows down the heart and diverts blood away from the muscles towards other system-maintenance processes. The two branches of the autonomic nervous system are so different that activating them together would be like accelerating and braking simultaneously.

The endocrine contribution to arousal also involves the adrenal glands (so called because they sit above each kidney), but it works more slowly than the sympathetic nervous system, taking minutes rather than a fraction of a second. The chemical signals from the hypothalamus (in the brain), relayed by the pituitary gland (just under the brain) cause the glands to release cortisol into the bloodstream. This is termed the 'hypothalamic-pituitary-adrenal axis' (HPA axis). Cortisol is a central stress hormone. To make energy available, it increases blood sugar (glucose) levels by counteracting the effects of insulin in order to release fatty acid from the body's stores of fat. In the brain it increases vigilance, backing up the effects of adrenaline. In addition, the pituitary gland releases several other hormones during stress, including prolactin – which inhibits reproductive processes – and morphine-like pain-killers, some of which are also produced by the brain. Much of this makes obvious sense in an evolved adaptive strategy whereby short-term emergencies take priority.

Other physiological responses to stress include the inhibition of growth hormone and reproductive hormones such as oestrogen, progesterone and testosterone, as well as the inhibition of insulin. These responses all ensure that energy is kept for use instead of being stored for future needs. Sustained stress also disrupts various aspects of the immune system, mainly through the HPA axis but also through the activation of the sympathetic nervous system. In the short term (within the first hour of stress) the immune response seems to be enhanced but prolonged stress seriously weakens it. One common tendency is for high levels of cortisol to shrink the thymus gland, thereby halting the production of new lymphocytes (the white blood cells of the immune system). This effect is so reliable that the size of the thymus gland was sometimes used as an indication of cortisol levels before this hormone could easily be measured directly.

Serious consequences for health arise when anxiety and physiological arousal are sustained or recur frequently over weeks, months or years. The feedback mechanisms – which should return the systems to normal – can be damaged by sustained periods of arousal. The regulation of cortisol is an example. The nerve cells in the hippocampus that provide the feedback for the regulation of cortisol become damaged by excessive cortisol. Their numbers decrease during ageing, a process accelerated by chronic arousal. This means that the feedback mechanism controlling cortisol is blunted and resting levels creep slowly upwards over the years. It also means that in brief emergencies cortisol responses are blunted: instead of reaching a brief peak and then rapidly falling back to normal when the emergency is over, cortisol levels rise more slowly and take longer to return to what has become a higher normal baseline. This has the makings of a vicious circle that ratchets up the resting cortisol levels throughout an individual's life.

Similar processes probably contribute to the upward

regulation of several other systems involved in physiological arousal, including the age-related increase in blood pressure and blood clotting time, but the evidence is less clear. Although stress leads to a transient increase in blood pressure, the link between this and the increase in blood pressure with age remains to be convincingly demonstrated. Nevertheless, the increase in blood pressure with age does seem to be related to social changes associated with long-term economic development: it is absent in pre-agricultural societies but becomes increasingly apparent in successive stages of economic development. In addition, blood pressure was found not to rise with age in one closed monastic order. As well as the increase in resting levels, blood pressure can also show the pattern of blunted responses to short-term stress found for cortisol among the chronically stressed.

The effect of chronic anxiety on immunity may also be part of a related pattern. Because overactivation of the immune system leads to autoimmune diseases, in which the body's defence mechanisms are triggered unnecessarily, the initial heightened immune responses during short-term stress would be dangerous if prolonged. Sapolsky suggests that the dampening secondary effect of cortisol on the immune system may have evolved to ensure that immune responses are quickly returned to normal. When arousal is sustained for long periods, however, these secondary effects can substantially suppress the immune system, thereby increasing the risks of infectious disease. Note that infectious agents are now thought to contribute to the initiation or promotion of several diseases – including coronary heart diseases and some cancers – not normally regarded as infectious in themselves.

Chronic stress can also damage the mechanism by which insulin controls the concentration of glucose in the blood. As cortisol is an insulin antagonist, increased levels cause specialized receptors on fat cells to become less sensitive to the insulin signal to store energy – so keeping high levels of energy available in circulation.

The accumulated physiological impact of chronic stress has been called 'allostatic load'. Its indications are higher blood pressure, insulin resistance, central obesity and raised basal cortisol levels. The higher the load, the greater the risks of cardiovascular disease, cancer and infection, and the faster the decline in mental functioning in old age (because the hippocampus, which is central to learning and memory, is very sensitive to cortisol). A particularly important disease pathway involves the rapid clogging of the arteries, which can lead to heart attack. If the energy resources mobilized during physiological arousal – in the form of fatty acids released from fat tissue into the bloodstream – are not used in the physical activity of fight or flight, then they are likely to increase the cholesterol deposits that clog the arteries. Sustained inactivity and anxiety add to the risks of cardiovascular disease. So increased allostatic load may contribute to disease through several different pathways.

Ageing and increased allostatic load have features in common. As the effects of chronic stress appear to increase the wear and tear of some biological systems, they have been likened to more rapid ageing. And just as ageing increases the risk of a wide range of diseases, so too does chronic anxiety. As a 'general vulnerability' factor, chronic anxiety would help explain why such a wide range of diseases are more common among lower socioeconomic groups. (The existence of a 'general vulnerability' factor such as chronic stress does not of course mean that there are not other important disease-specific contributions.)

Another aspect of chronic anxiety that is relevant to explaining the socioeconomic gradient in health concerns the timing of its effects. The health gradient is built up of three different kinds of influences during life: people's current circumstances, the cumulative effects of experiences over a lifetime, and the effects of the early childhood and prenatal environments. Stress too works through these three different patterns. Lifelong arousal and stress responses are influenced, as we shall see, by exposure to prenatal and postnatal stress and early emotional development. In addition, the biological processes through which chronic anxiety increases vulnerability to ill-health are clearly cumulative over long stretches of life. Finally, there are also processes linking current stress to more immediate health risks such as the increased risk of infection or blood clots.

These processes would make perfect evolutionary sense where the survival advantages of a more effective response to short-term emergencies outweighed the small long-term health costs. The health costs would be substantial only where stresses were maintained for long periods – something that was probably uncommon among our prehistoric ancestors. But perhaps not all the effects of chronic anxiety are simply the harmful costs of biological responses to emergencies. In dominance hierarchies, low-status animals do seem to suffer chronic anxiety. To survive in more dangerous circumstances, with frequent threats of attack, it would be adaptive if there were an upward regulation of resting levels of arousal so that the

43

body was readier at any moment to respond to threats – permanently more ready to fight or flee.

Stress responses may be particularly sensitive to conditions in early life. Studies in humans and animals indicate that prenatal and postnatal stress has powerful effects on anxiety levels and stress responses, and that these effects can last throughout much of later life. In people and animals who suffer emotional stress early in life, blood pressure and cortisol levels increase faster with age. As the epidemiologist Clyde Hertzman and others have argued, this kind of early programming is probably related to the way in which early emotional development – poor attachment – seems to cast a long shadow forwards over health in later life.

There are likely to be advantages if the settings of some of the stress responses and the state of physiological preparedness were initially sensitive to the different kinds of society, or positions within a society, into which a child might be born. For many years psychologists have drawn attention to the importance of early emotional experience and the lifelong effects of insecure emotional attachment. The psychiatrist John Bowlby believed that the evolutionary explanation of the importance of secure early emotional attachment was that it ensured that an infant sought the security of its mother's protection when faced with danger; but that does not explain why early emotional attachment has lifelong effects. With the benefit of evidence from studies of humans and several other mammalian species, however, we are now left in little doubt that prenatal and postnatal social experiences probably regulate not only the child's autonomic nervous system but also the HPA axis. This early programming gives rise to different levels of stress hormones and emotional reactivity throughout much of later life. Rather than simply seeing secure attachment as good, and insecure attachment as bad, it is reasonable to view the increased anxiety and aggressiveness as adaptive to more conflictual social environments.

People often seek to explain the long-term effects of early emotional life by suggesting that our relationship as adults to wider authority in society is modelled on our childhood relationship to parental authority. But this view is probably partly misconceived. In our evolutionary past, the nuclear family and the wider society would not usually have existed as two separate social environments. Instead, children would have been brought up within a small, closely integrated, probably nomadic group of adults. There would not have been the same contrast between the world of the private family and a wider, anonymous, large-scale society. In addition to its parents, a child in our evolutionary past would know, and be known by, a number of other adults. A child's development would be less a matter of transferring a relationship from the family to society at large than a more continuous experience of growing up in an extended social group. This would have been true not only of the hunter-gatherer bands, but also of the small territorial groups of our pre-human forebears. So rather than early social learning and stress responses being transferred perhaps inappropriately from the nuclear family to the wider society, our ancestors would have experienced a less discontinuous social environment.

Interestingly, it now looks as if postnatal emotional stress has many of the same effects as prenatal stress. In humans, not only are fetal and maternal levels of cortisol correlated during pregnancy, but babies' cortisol levels are associated with maternal stress during pregnancy. These connections have been confirmed by findings from animal experiments. Pregnant female rats exposed experimentally to stress had young offspring with increased cortisol and anxiety levels. What is more, the effects on the young could be blocked by drugs interfering with the effects of anxiety on cortisol production. These links between maternal stress and the welfare of the next generation are all the more important because they are likely to explain a substantial part of the relationship between birthweight (more particularly body length at birth) and the incidence of some diseases in later life. The epidemiologist David Barker has shown that people who were small as babies are more likely to develop a range of conditions including heart disease, stroke and insulin resistance and to show signs of more rapid ageing. In animal experiments, maternal stress in infancy leads to reduced birthweight; and the programming of the HPA axis in early life provides a plausible link with later disease.

Given that our social environments can differ so radically, it would make good sense if the arousal mechanism (the HPA axis) were responsive to early social experience. Different kinds of society require very different social strategies. Different patterns of arousal and emotional responsiveness will be appropriate, depending on whether a child grows up in a sharing, egalitarian group, in which cooperative behaviour and reciprocity are rewarded, or whether it finds itself in a competitive group, in which social dominance and an ability to fend for oneself are everything. Using the right strategy is clearly crucial. The use of affiliative strategies in a dominance hierarchy is likely to lead to exploitation rather than reciprocity. The use of dominance strategies in an affiliative group is likely to lead to exclusion from the cooperative group. Appropriately, higher cortisol levels seem to be associated with more aggressive and less affiliative behaviour.

We can now see that secure early emotional attachment and the transmission of prenatal stress from mother to fetus are important in preparing the child for the kind of society and social relationships that it will have to deal with. It is tempting to view a secure early life within the protective fold of a loving nuclear family as setting us up with the basic confidence to meet the challenges of the wider society. Instead, it appears that in our evolutionary past, early social experience would have served as a taster for the kind of society in which we would have to live. It is likely that the basic form of social organization in small nomadic groups would have had some long-term stability.

Early programming of stress responses might also make evolutionary sense if it prepared individuals for responses appropriate to their social rank. Here the key element may have been height. Studies of child development suggest that early growth may be compromised by prenatal and postnatal stress. In addition, small children are less likely to move up in society. As a result of the influence of early stress on growth, being small in childhood is highly predictive of increased cortisol level and blood pressure later in life. In modern society, people who are tall – particularly those who were tall as children – are much more likely to move up the social ladder, as the biologist Scott Montgomery has shown. This is probably because people who are tall as children (that is, tall after allowing

47

for inherited influences on height) are tall because they have had an emotionally secure early childhood and are more socially confident and able as adults. In troops of animals where size is an important determinant of position on the dominance hierarchy, factors compromising growth are predictive of low social status. These factors also help to prepare the emotional responses for the constant vigilance needed by subordinate animals if they are to survive.

Even if some of these mechanisms were appropriate to prehistoric conditions, they are often a disadvantage in modern life. An example is the way in which stress makes the blood clot more easily. When facing imminent physical danger and risk of wounding, it is important that the blood should clot quickly in order to minimize blood loss. This is achieved by increases in the clotting factor, fibrinogen, in response to increased adrenaline produced during stress. In monkeys the most common attacks are by dominant animals on subordinates. But higher fibrinogen levels are also more common in junior office staff, as if their subordinate positions put them at risk of physical attack from their superiors. Increased fibrinogen levels seem to be one of the contributors to the much higher rates of heart attack in junior staff than in senior staff. If we lived in a social environment in which there was a constant threat of *physical* attack by superiors, the costs – in terms of increased risk of heart attack – of maintaining permanently higher fibrinogen levels could easily be outweighed by the decreased risk of blood loss in the event of injury. Our knowledge of the social gradient in fibrinogen comes principally from the Whitehall Study which followed up 10,000 civil servants. Interestingly, the same study also points to the importance of being able to control your work. It seems likely that one reason why control is important is that in the context of office work it represents autonomy, and its opposite is probably more supervision and subordination.

Sapolsky tells two stories that illustrate both the evolutionary age of some of these mechanisms and their relevance to health inequalities among humans. Although most of the biological responses to stress that we have mentioned appear to be common among mammalian species, some of them are much older than others. Consider the death of salmon shortly after spawning. The biological mechanisms that lead to death involve very high concentrations of cortisol. Sapolsky says that salmon caught after spawning 'have huge adrenal glands, peptic ulcers, and kidney lesions; their immune systems have collapsed and they are teaming with parasites and infections'. Because their system for regulating cortisol seems to break down during spawning, these fish have extraordinarily high concentrations of cortisol. But are their ills really due simply to increased levels of cortisol? Apparently they are: if their adrenal glands are removed after spawning so cortisol concentrations cannot increase, the fish do not die. This mechanism is not only found in five species of salmon; it has also evolved independently among several species of Australian marsupial mice in which the males die soon after mating. The same mechanisms are at work: they too survive if their adrenal glands are removed.

Sapolsky's second story concerns the effects of chronic stress on paupers. When, early in the twentieth century, medical students learned their anatomy by dissecting the bodies of paupers, they became accustomed to seeing adrenal glands of a certain size. But when middle-class people started to leave their bodies for medical education and research, anatomists began to see much smaller adrenal glands. Assuming that there was something wrong with the smaller ones, they named the mysterious condition 'idiopathic adrenal atrophy'. Only later did it become clear that the abnormal adrenal glands were those belonging to paupers, presumably enlarged as a result of the chronic stress associated with living in poverty.

CHAPTER 4

....

Social Comparison,
Social Anxiety and Conclusions

We have seen how hierarchical social relations and social position influence health. We have also seen that matters of status and respect are a key component of violence. In addition, the various relationships between health and both income and income inequality highlight the importance of relative income. Both Adam Smith and Karl Marx, in common with most of today's authorities, define poverty in relative terms (the European Union defines poverty as the condition of living on less than half the national average income). Smith and several modern economists also emphasize the powerful contribution that hierarchical social comparisons make to the desire for higher incomes and consumption.

The ability to make social comparisons, at least in terms of judgements of relative strength and social rank, must be part of the survival skills of any animal that needs to avoid fruitless and dangerous conflicts in a dominance hierarchy. Indeed, the most primitive source of social comparison may have been the need in any social species to assess the strength of other individuals relative to one's own. Such social comparisons are clearly part of the instinctive equipment of many animal species. But social comparisons among humans go much deeper.

As reflexive beings, we know ourselves partly through the eyes of others. As we monitor ourselves in relation to others, part of our experience of ourselves is our imagined view of how others see us. This ability is one of the foundations of human social life and close to the core of what we mean when we call ourselves 'social beings'. As well as the value of well-tuned social antennae that enable us to shape our social behaviour in relation to others' reactions to us, it is also likely that social comparisons are a precondition for cultural integration and learning. Without detailed social comparison and self-monitoring, it is difficult to see how a child could acquire language. Most informal learning must involve processes of imitation and self-correction. Even when not related to social hierarchy, these processes would seem to involve evaluative judgements of whether one's practice is adequate or inadequate, better or worse, successful or unsuccessful.

Charles Darwin, whose book *The Expression of the Emotions in Man and Animals* has a chapter on blushing entitled 'Self-attention, Shame, Shyness, Modesty' in which he argues that shame 'depends in all cases on . . . a sensitive regard for the opinion, more particularly the depreciation of others'. The eminent psychologist Thomas Scheff sees shame as a more broadly based kind of social anxiety than the term itself suggests. He views it as playing a fundamental role in social conformity and obedience to authority. When we talk about having low self-esteem, or feeling foolish, stupid, ridiculous, inadequate, defective, incompetent, awkward, exposed, vulnerable, insecure or helpless, we are, he says, talking about shameful experiences that are involved in the social process of monitoring self in the eyes of others. Indeed, Darwin pointed out that we feel shame, embarrassment and shyness particularly in the presence of 'equals and superiors', of those we 'revere'. Emphasizing the intimate link between shame and social status, Paul Gilbert and Michael McGuire say that 'Shame is nearly always associated with depictions of loss of status . . . of being devalued, disgraced, demoted, and dishonoured.' Scheff regards shame as part of what he calls the 'deference-emotion system', and Darwin draws attention to the fact that in several languages the words for shyness and for fear are closely related. As if to complement Darwin's observation that even shy people 'are rarely shy in the presence of those with whom they are quite familiar, and of whose good opinion and sympathy they are perfectly assured', Gilbert emphasizes how feelings of shame are related to 'processing socially threatening information – particularly in the domains of social rank/status and social exclusions/rejection'.

In the context of the equality of prehistoric hunter-gatherers, it is worth noting that although, as Darwin points out, shame and embarrassment most often result when we have committed some social *faux pas*, people also feel embarrassed when they are too strongly praised. If 'counter-dominance strategies' were the basis of primitive equity, as Christopher Boehm and others have suggested, then undue social prominence was perhaps better avoided.

The capacity for shame, or at least shamefaced behaviour, is widespread in social mammals – indeed, it is hard not to give anthropomorphic interpretations to a dog's cringing posture when its owners express anger at its wrong-doing. Gilbert and McGuire have argued that the capacity for shame is crucial to the functioning of dominance hierarchies. Because dominance hierarchies are essentially power hierarchies, the only way in which subordinate animals can avoid endless dangerous and fruitless conflict is to meet dominance behaviour with submissiveness. As Gilbert and McGuire say:

> Shame signals (e.g. head down, gaze avoidance, and hiding) are generally regarded as submissive and appeasement displays, designed to de-escalate and/or escape from conflict. Thus insofar as shame is related to submissiveness and appeasement behaviour, then it is a damage limitation strategy, adopted when continuing in a shameless, nonsubmissive way might provoke very serious attacks or rejections from others.

Allan Schore argues that the shame response develops towards the end of the first year of life with the growth of the prefrontal cortex of the brain, which is dependent on the interaction between parent and child. Soon after the infant has become used to pleasurable attention and eye contact during the first year, parents start shaping the child's behaviour through expressions of disapproval. The pleasurable face-to-face interactions of attachment are frequently replaced by the caregiver's expressions of disgust. Indeed, Helen Lewis called shame the 'attachment emotion'. If this is the basis of the early programming of the HPA axis, it is not hard to imagine the effects of much higher levels of stress, including that resulting from anger and domestic conflict.

Thomas Scheff gives examples of the importance of shame in both social conformity and obedience to authority. He discusses Solomon Asch's 1952 experiments, which demonstrated that subjects would go along with prevailing group opinion rather than make their own independent judgement of which of two lines shown on a screen is the same length as a third. The subjects later reported that they went along with prevailing opinion for fear of looking stupid, or because others might think they 'couldn't see straight'. On voluntary obedience to authority, Scheff discusses Stanley Milgram's 1969 experiments in which people voluntary administered what they were led to believe were very painful and even life-threatening electric shocks to students in what they took to be a 'learning experiment' – all for no better reason than that a supervisor told them that the shocks were a necessary part of the experiment.

So how do all these findings relate to health and the identification of the most powerful sources of chronic anxiety related to low social status? The literature on shame should probably not be treated separately from a much wider body of work on *social anxiety*, most of which centres on 'evaluation anxiety'. The 'social anxiety' literature embraces work on what is perhaps most accurately called fear of negative social evaluation, and brings into its orbit work on shyness, embarrassment, 'behavioural inhibition', 'fear of failure', 'approval motivation', 'self-conscious affect', 'interpersonal competence' and 'sense of inferiority' or 'inferiority complex'. It concentrates on the anxieties that arise from how we are seen by others, and so encompasses shame, disrespect, invidious social comparisons, desire for social status or 'regard', desire for acceptance and fear of rejection by friends and so on.

The psychologists Mark Leary and Robin Kowalski have tried to unify some slightly different evolutionary explanations of the capacity for shame. They write:

> We favor the idea that social anxiety evolved as a mechanism for fostering social inclusion and minimizing the possibility of rejection or exclusion ... The most parsimonious evolutionary explanation of social anxiety is that it evolved as a mechanism for fostering and maintaining one's membership in supportive (i.e. mutually interdependent) groups and relationships.

Central to these social anxieties are processes of social comparison, fears of inferiority and inadequacy in relation to others. According to the psychologist Peter Trower and colleagues, 'socially anxious people ... perceive themselves as subordinates in hostile hierarchies and utilize submissiveness and other "reverted escape" behaviors to minimise loss of status and rejection.' Leary and Kowalski's 'sociometer theory' holds that maintaining self-esteem involves monitoring our behaviour and other people's reception of it for indications of social disapproval or rejection. In this way, our behaviour can be corrected when signs of rejection are detected. In short, 'the self-esteem system may have evolved as a mechanism for minimising the likelihood of social exclusion.'

As well as showing us why we are so sensitive to social comparisons, the work on social anxiety and shame indicates some of the experiential implications of, and behavioural responses to, social comparisons in the context of inequality. It also casts more light on the reasons why patterns of violence and friendship are also part of the nexus of chronic anxiety and health.

We saw in Chapter 1 that violence is related to income inequality in much the same way that health is, and that the distributions of violence and of death from non-violent causes are closely related. As the shared etymology of the words 'anxiety' and 'anger' suggests, social anxiety and violence have common origins. Scheff points to the link between shame and anger, saying that 'hostility can be viewed as an attempt to ward off feelings of humiliation generated by inept, ineffectual moves, and by a sense of incompetence, insults, and a lack of power to defend against insults.' He sees a 'shame–rage spiral' as part of what he calls the 'deference emotion system'. 'As humilia-tion increases,' he writes, 'rage and hostility increase proportionally to defend against loss of self-esteem.' Others have also suggested that anger may be a response to shame. Gilbert describes how covering shame with anger is a 'face-saving' strategy and a frequent source of male violence.

We have already seen how violence is related to people's feelings that they are not respected. In clarifying the relationships between violence, disrespect and social status, Scheff describes how pride – the opposite of shame – arises from deferential treatment and signs of respect from others, whereas shame reflects lack of respect and deference. In a shaming situation we have a choice of either behaving deferentially and accepting the lack of respect, or denying it and attempting to force others to respect us.

In this context, it would be easy to assume that shame would just give rise to meek and deferential behaviour; but it is important to recognize that shame is just as closely related to the violent rejection of the disparaging look or gesture and the inferiority it implies. The increased cortisol concentrations produced by states of high anxiety are just as much a preparation for fight as for flight. Violence is often a defence against threatened loss of respect or status.

Social anxiety also contributes to the important relationship between friendship and health. Research findings seem to confirm that the more anxious, shy or insecure people are, the less likely they are to have the confidence to initiate social contact and the more likely they are to withdraw from it. Leary and Kowalski conclude that people who feel socially anxious tend to *disaffiliate*: their less sociable behaviour is a form of avoidance linked specifically to social anxiety. Socially anxious people report less contact with friends, have fewer casual conversations and are less likely to initiate conversations. In addition, they apparently have shorter conversations, speak more quietly and engage in less eye contact with other people: nevertheless, they wish they could participate more fully in social encounters. Interestingly, this disaffiliation is a specific response to *social* anxiety – to other people as the source of anxiety: when facing a non-social source of anxiety, such as a hospital visit for minor surgery, people naturally prefer friends to be with them.

The relationship between social anxiety and friendship is, however, a two-way interaction. Although social anxieties tend to reduce social affiliation, there is no doubt that friendship also reduces social anxiety. Feeling liked and appreciated is obviously an important source of reassurance that feeds into positive self-evaluation. There is also likely to be a two-way relationship between social anxiety on the one hand, and social cohesion and the quality of the social environment on the other hand. Not only will smaller inequalities in income and social status tend to reduce social anxiety in a population and thus make people more socially confident, but improved norms of social interaction and a more supportive and inclusive social environment will also feed back to reduce social anxiety more widely.

There are, of course, important sex differences in response to anxiety. While men are much more likely to be violent, recent research by Shelley Taylor suggests that women are more likely to seek the security of friends and social affiliations. But this is far from the confident, outgoing, affiliative behaviour that fosters social cohesion. Social anxiety is the enemy of wider social affiliations.

In terms of the causal pathways affecting health, social cohesion may be regarded almost as an epiphenomenon. Despite the statistical associations, it is clearly implausible to think that saying 'hello' to neighbours or going to an occasional meeting of some club or voluntary association can do wonders for your health. What affects health is the individual experience of chronic stress arising from social anxiety. Social cohesion is associated with health because it is a reflection of how tense or relaxed social contacts are, and of the underlying social anxiety. So saying 'hello' to neighbours and belonging to local groups are related to health because they are indicative of lower levels of anxiety. The only sense in which social cohesion is not an epiphenomenon is through feedback effects as improved social interaction leads to feelings of being accepted and further reductions in social anxiety.

Finally, depression is also linked to social anxiety: it is, as Leary and Kowalski say, the most common emotional manifestation of social anxiety. Just as the shame response may be a form of appeasement, Gilbert argues that depression arises from psychological processes that have evolved from responses related to defeat and submission. Without it, dominance behaviour would – as we said earlier – lead to continuous conflict, so the capacity to submit and accept subordinate status has survival value. Depression may therefore result from a sense of defeat and failure in a situation you cannot escape. When you are unable to control the situation, and the possibilities of fight or flight are both blocked, a depressed mind-set (consisting of low self-evaluation and acceptance of defeat or being a failure), which leads people to present themselves as downcast, unchallenging and unthreatening, would at least mean they avoided further dangerous and fruitless conflict. If it had no such survival value, it seems unlikely that we would be so prone to such an incapacitating condition as serious depression.

Gilbert lists the various kinds of situation known to cause depression in which people feel defeated and devalued, and suffer setbacks and loss of control. He also emphasizes that in humans the sense of being defeated, of having failed, does not usually come from direct involvement in social conflict. Rather, it may involve a wide range of areas invoking feelings of competence and incompetence – from insoluble family problems to failure to win promotion – in which the depressed person makes 'unfavourable judgements about their relative rank . . . their attractiveness, talents, competencies, desirability to others or "power" '. As Gilbert says, low self-confidence is affected by unfavourable social comparisons and can be seen as 'involuntary subordinate self perception.'

Towards a better society

The picture we are left with reflects the importance of the social environment in human evolution. As we noted earlier, good relationships with other people have always been crucial to human welfare – even to our basic material welfare. Indeed, several modern theories of the evolution of the human brain maintain that the principal selective environmental stimulus to its rapid growth may have been the demands of having to deal with the complexity of social life. Rather than thinking of the human brain as having developed simply to deal with problems of the material environment, we need to think of it much more as a social organ. To understand our apparent sensitivity to social status and friendship, we need to view the brain not as having generalized computing power, but as having modules for dealing with particular aspects of social life in much the same way as it has modules for language acquisition or for facial recognition. However, abandoning the view of the brain as generalized computing power and recognizing that it has an evolved attentiveness to particular aspects of social life does not mean that the environment in general, or the social environment in particular, is a less important determinant of behaviour. Instead, it gives us a clearer idea of how the environment affects behaviour. The extent of our desire for friends and concern for social status does not rigidly determine how friendly, egalitarian or hierarchical our societies are. Nevertheless, recognition of the deep-seated nature of these desires and concerns may increase our understanding of the problems of different social systems and help us to improve the quality of our social environment.

We have seen that as income inequality increases, the quality of the social environment seems to deteriorate: trust decreases, involvement in local community life decreases and hostility and violence increase. In other words, as hierarchical dominance becomes stronger, egalitarian social relationships weaken. Friendship and low social status are strongly associated with health and strongly associated (inversely) with each other, because they represent two sides of the same coin. They are in effect the two opposite bases of human association: either through affiliative strategies, or through strategies based on dominance, power, and its counterpart – submission. The weakening of affiliative social relationships may be partly due to a shift in people's choice of social strategy as they find themselves facing a social reality in which power and the hierarchical dimension have become predominant. The name of the game changes as the balance of advantage between affiliative and dominance strategies shifts. Perhaps simultaneously more children are brought up exposed to greater conflict, programmed with increased anxiety, and readier for fight or flight, but less likely to use affiliative social strategies.

Given the link with social anxiety, inequality may have become more important during the historical development of individualism and the disappearance of stable communities in which people tended to know, and be known by, the same people throughout their lives. In geographically and socially mobile mass societies, in which social status is acquired rather than ascribed, and in which we constantly encounter people we have never met before, there is a growing concern with self-presentation. This suggests that we have become more prone to anxieties about social evaluation.

Psychology has a vast literature on the insecurities and fears of inadequacy associated with emotional development in early childhood, and remarkably little on social stratification. Sociology is the mirror image of this situation: it has a vast literature on the effects of social status and social stratification, and little on emotional development in early childhood. But there can be little doubt that personal insecurity from early childhood makes people more vulnerable to the insecurities and fears of inadequacy associated with low social status. The social hierarchy all too often appears as if it were an ordering of success and ability, from the most capable at the top, to the most incapable at the bottom. Differing incomes, social status, and levels of inequality affect the stresses of family life. Children are brought up with quite different experiences of attachment and conflict which prepare them to use different social strategies and cope with qualitatively different social environments in adulthood. Dominance relations are more stressful and incur health costs that go with greater physiological arousal and anxiety.

The social anxiety explanation of the power of social risk factors (low social status, weak social affiliations, and prenatal and postnatal stress) does more than provide a plausible account of their otherwise inexplicable strength. It also explains some of the links with violence and other measures of the social environment. It does so by suggesting that social anxieties are triggered by evolved sensitivities to aspects of our social environment that would have been important to survival and reproductive success in our evolutionary past. We can be confident that they affect health through chronic anxiety because evidence from non-human primates, and increasingly from human beings, shows that these social risk factors are all associated with higher baseline cortisol levels.

This book has concentrated on the psychosocial pathways linking socioeconomic circumstances to health, not because material factors affect health only through psychosocial pathways, but because these pathways seem to provide the most important link between the two. Although the pathways probably have the greatest influence on our quality of life, they are also the least well understood. The evidence suggests that smoking, heavy alcohol consumption and eating for comfort may also be responses to anxiety. Because alcohol and drugs reduce social inhibitions they are often used to deal with social anxieties. In so far as these and other behavioural risk factors are related to social anxiety, they are likely to contribute to the same patterns.

More affiliative strategies that foster social solidarity are unlikely to prevail without more egalitarian economic underpinnings. In the developed world, as much as half of the variation in population health, in homicide rates and in social cohesion appears to be due to differences in income inequality alone. Although there are many other influences, inequality is a crucially important part of the picture. Nor is this picture based on an unrealistic contrast between the levels of inequality common in modern societies and some unreachable level of total equality. Rather, the picture reflects the importance of the comparatively small differences in inequality between US states or between the developed market democracies. Perhaps the most exciting aspect of the emerging picture is that the psychosocial welfare of modern populations is not merely an individual variable, but is also deeply influenced by structural factors such as the extent of inequality.

The picture of the destructive effects of inequality that we have built up in the preceding pages contrasts with more familiar analyses of class and class conflict. Marx saw the classes themselves, as well as the nature of the conflict between them, as being constituted by their differing relations to the system of production – whether as slave owners and slaves, feudal lords and serfs, or capitalists and workers. These qualitatively different relations were the cause of the conflict: they defined both the battleground and the parties to the conflict. But the analysis we have developed suggests that dominance hierarchies are a more fundamental source of conflict and social tension. In an important sense social inequality is the stuff of which class is made. Differences in people's relation to the production system might count for rather little if those differences were not given a social charge by being overlaid by inequalities in power and wealth, resulting in the view of one group as superior to the other. As well as class, other kinds of difference – such as those between ethnic, linguistic or religious groups – also become sources of tension when overlaid by inequality.

Emphasizing the costs of inequality itself is not to deny that class differences constituted through different types of relation to the production system have been crucially important in the past; but social and economic systems are constantly changing, and it is becoming increasingly important to distinguish between the effects of class and the effects of inequality. In the advanced developed societies today, most income comes from employment or self-employment, and most capital is institutional capital managed by banks, insurance companies, pension funds and other financial institutions. There are, of course, still people who live on profits or rent rather than on their own labour, and some of the capital invested on the stock market is still invested and managed by private individuals. Nevertheless, it is easy to imagine modern societies moving towards a system in which almost all income was earned and almost all capital was institutional capital managed by financial analysts employed to shift money around to maximize profits. In such a society there would be no class divisions based on distinctions such as those between owners and their employees. Yet if the scale of income differences remained as wide as it is now, there can be little doubt that such societies would feel much the same as ours: still characterized by racial prejudice, social exclusion, snobbery, elitism, violence and so on.

If the experience of living in an unequal but otherwise classless society would hardly differ from our experience of the current social reality, then it is the effects of inequality rather than of class that we need to analyse. We need to understand the effects of dominance hierarchies, of differences in income, status and power – of inequality itself.

The behavioural responses to dominance hierarchies include some of the nastiest features of discrimination and prejudice. When non-human primates in a dominance hierarchy lose a battle for status, they often show aggression towards others below them. This phenomenon is known in German as the *radfahrer-reaktion* (bicycling-reaction): having lost a battle, the animal bows to its superiors while kicking at those beneath it. The term originally came from Theodor Adorno's *Authoritarian Personality* (1950), which tried to explain the Nazis' treatment of Jews. We know that discrimination against vulnerable minorities and extreme nationalism increase in times of economic hardship: when unemployment is high, affected people may try to regain a sense of selfhood, status and respect by asserting their superiority over vulnerable ethnic and religious minorities; and in US states where income inequality is greater, racial prejudice is greater and there is more political and economic discrimination against women. Similarly, humiliated men are more likely to inflict violence on their wives. The underlying pattern is perhaps most clearly seen in the brutality shown towards sex offenders by fellow prisoners. These extremes are part of a continuum of dominance behaviour, from the use of subtle indicators of superiority and exclusiveness at the top, to overt violence and racism at the bottom. At every level, hierarchies are characterized by social exclusion rather than inclusion. That is why greater inequality is associated with a deterioration in the quality of social relations. But by understanding how inequality rules through its divisiveness, we can perhaps begin to reduce it and realize our common humanity.

The idea that the reduction in inequality would lead to slower economic growth is almost certainly false. There are now a number of empirical studies that show that greater equality is associated with faster, rather than slower, economic growth. One of the reasons why this relationship exists is, appropriately enough, that social capital is thought to improve economic efficiency. Excuses for governments to drag their feet over the reduction of inequality are thin on the ground. If we are to improve health and social capital, if we are to free ourselves of antisocial prejudices and create a more inclusive society, the reduction of inequalities must surely be a key political objective.

REFERENCES

Alexander, R. D. *The Biology of Moral Systems* (Aldine de Gruyter, New York, 1987).

Anzaldua, G., *Borderlands* (Aunt Lute Books, San Francisco, 1987).

Asch, S. E., *Social Psychology* (Prentice-Hall, Englewood Cliffs, 1952).

Barker, D. J. P., *Mothers, Babies and Health in Later Life*, 2nd edn (Churchill Livingstone, Edinburgh, 1998).

Bourdieu, P., *Distinction: A Social Critique of the Judgement of Taste* (Routledge, London, 1984).

Emerson, R. W., *The Conduct of Life* (Macmillan, London, 1883).

Erdal, D. and Whiten, A., Egalitarianism and Machiavellian intelligence in human evolution. In: *Modelling the Early Human Mind*, edited by Mellars, P. and Gibson, K. (McDonald Institute Monographs, Cambridge, 1996) 139–160.

Frank, R., *Luxury Fever* (Free Press, New York, 1999).

Gilbert, P., *Depression: The Evolution of Powerlessness* (Erlbaum, Hove, 1992).

Gilbert, P. and McGuire, M. T., Shame, status, and social roles: psychobiology and evolution. In: *Shame: Interpersonal Behavior, Psychopathology, and Culture,* edited by Gilbert, P. and Andrews, B. (Oxford University Press, 1998) 99–125.

Gilligan, J., *Violence: Our Deadly Epidemic and Its Causes* (Jessica Kingsley, London, 1999).

Jolly, A., *The Evolution of Primate Behavior* (Macmillan, New York, 1985).

Kawachi, I., Kennedy, B. and Wilkinson, R. G. (editors) *Income Inequality and Health*. Society and Population Health Reader vol. 1 (New Press, New York, 1999).

Keating, D. P. and Hertzman, C., *Development, Health and The Wealth of Nations: Social, Biological and Educational Dynamics* (Guilford Press, New York, 1999).

Leary, M. R. and Kowalski, R. M., *Social Anxiety* (Guilford Press, New York, 1995).

Leitenberg, H. (editor) *Handbook of Social and Evaluation Anxiety* (Plenum Press, New York, 1990).

Lewis, H. B., *Shame and Guilt in Neurosis* (International Universities Press, New York, 1971).

Marmot, M. G. and Wilkinson, R. G., *The Social Determinants of Health* (Oxford University Press, Oxford, 1999).

McCall, N., *Makes Me Wanna Holler: A Young Black Man in America* (Random House, New York, 1994).

Milgram, S., *Obedience to Authority* (Harper, New York, 1969).

Montgomery, S. M., Bartley, M. J., Cook, D. G. and Wadsworth, M. E. J., Health and social precursors of unemployment in young men in Great Britain. *Journal of Epidemiology and Community Health* 1996; 50(4): 415–422.

Putnam, R. D., Leonardi, R. and Nanatti, R. Y., *Making Democracy Work: Civic Traditions in Modern Italy* (Princeton University Press, 1993).

Sapolsky, R. M., *Why Zebras Don't Get Ulcers: A Guide to Stress, Stress-related Disease and Coping*, 2nd edn (Freeman, New York, 1998).

Scheff, T. J., *Microsociology: Discourse, Emotion and Social Structure* (University of Chicago Press, 1990).

Schor, J., *The Overspent American: When Buying Becomes You* (Basic Books, New York, 1998).

Trower, P., Gilbert, P. and Sherling, G., Social anxiety, evolution and self-presentation. In: *Handbook of Social and Evaluation Anxiety*, edited by Leitenberg, H. (Plenum Press, New York, 1990) 11–45.

Wilkinson, R. G., *Unhealthy Societies: The Afflictions of Inequality* (Routledge, London, 1996).